Omornah, Sr.

For a most special Carole!

_4-24-04_

THE REAL
Angels Among Us

PHIL SMART SR.

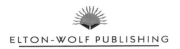
ELTON-WOLF PUBLISHING

Cover design by Jamie O'Neill
Text design by Jamie O'Neill

Cover photograph © Don Hammond/CORBIS

Text and pictures provided by Phil Smart Sr.
All rights to text and pictures reserved by author and may not be reproduced without permission.

Published by Elton-Wolf Publishing
Seattle, Washington

ISBN: 1-58619-102-0
Library of Congress Catalogue Number: 2003114996

08 07 06 05 04   1 2 3 4 5

First Edition February 2004

Printed in Canada

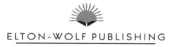

ELTON-WOLF PUBLISHING
2505 Second Avenue Suite 515 Seattle, Washington 98121
Tel 206.748.0345 Fax 206.748.0343
www.elton-wolf.com info@elton-wolf.com

What would you do if you knew you had time in the week to make a difference in the world?

A candle loses nothing by lighting another candle.

—Erin Majors

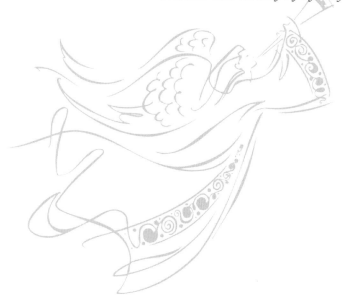

*M*any years ago, Phil Smart Sr. made time in his crowded schedule for a five-minute appointment that changed his life forever. The receptionist at his dealership, Phil Smart Mercedes Benz, said to him one morning, "There's a woman in the lobby waiting to see you. She says her name is 'Grandma Christmas Card.'"

"With a name like that," Phil recalls, "I knew she had to be in marketing."

Her real name was Peg Emery, a volunteer with Children's Hospital, and within a few minutes she had persuaded the car dealer to buy several dozen engraved Christmas cards to support the hospital's work. But Peg wasn't through. A few days later she returned to Phil's office with a personal invitation.

"Since the hospital was founded in 1907, we've never had a man volunteer his time in the evenings to visit our young patients. The all-woman board of directors would like you to be that person. It would just be three hours one night a week. Will you do it?"

"Where is the manual for male volunteers?" Phil asked.

"We don't have one," said Peg. "Once you meet the children you won't need any instructions."

With no formal training on how to comfort critically ill children, and after assuring his wife Helen that it would mean just three hours one night a week, Phil said yes to Peg Emery's invitation.

That initial visit turned into three visits, and then six months of visits, and then a year. Soon, a lifetime of giving to others unfolded with no expectation other than the opportunity to share himself with the children who have taught him what life is all about.

For the past forty-two years, every Wednesday night Phil has been able to go to this place he calls the miracle house, Children's Hospital and Regional Medical Center.

It's been the school where Phil has learned about life. Every visit, every child has become a precious gift, unwrapped before him.

There was Bonnie, who as a ten-year-old could move only her head and tongue, but who found a way to earn both a bachelor's and master's degree in counseling so she could help drug addicts in her hometown get back on their feet.

And there was Jeff, who met Phil thirty-three years ago. Jeff came to the miracle house to recover from a catastrophic injury. Today, he, too, is a ward volunteer.

One day the hospital called and offered Phil what he refers to as a promotion. They asked him to donate more of his time. When he asked, "How much more time?" the voice on the other end of the line said, "Not much, just one additional day a year. We'll give you a new suit for the job but you might not like the color. It's all red."

Phil took his new job to heart and soon became affectionately known as "the real Santa Claus."

Phil is eighty-four years old now. He has been a ward volunteer for more than half his life. If ever there was a real Santa Claus, who understands the gift of giving, you will find him at the miracle house every Wednesday night.

Phil has had the privilege to know each of these children by name. He has shared their hospital hopes and fears. They have shown him the one thing in life he could never have understood on his own: how a little time invested in another person can transform your heart and change the world.

This is a lesson Phil had already learned as a Scoutmaster and past president of the Chief Seattle Council, and as a forty-one-year member and past president of Seattle "4" Rotary, the largest rotary club in the world when he was its president fourteen years ago.

When he reports in for his weekly visits, some of the young patients call him "the angel from heaven." Phil chuckles and says, "I've never heard a car dealer called that before!"

While this book tells his stories in print, Phil often speaks with large groups. Invariably, one question always arises from the audience: "How do you run a business, deal with the demands of daily life, and find time to volunteer?"

He smiles and says, "I've been given as much time as anyone else: eight hours to work, eight hours to sleep, and eight hours to spend as I please. It's out of this third eight that I've become a changed person. The children at the hospital have molded me into a happier man."

By this time, Phil's audience is leaning forward as if to say, "Tell me more."

He is grateful to oblige. He shares the stories of his young "teachers" with his audience, hoping that a bit of his vision will rub off on them. Some are wiping their eyes. Some are smiling. All are listening.

—Mark Cutshall

About Children's Hospital

Bill Gates Sr.

The author of this book has enriched his life through his service to children. In doing so, he becomes a representative of the legions of individuals who have, for nearly a hundred years now, given a piece of their lives and the whole of their hearts to Children's Hospital. They include volunteers, Board and Guild members, fundraisers for hospital events, and contributors to Children's in a million different ways.

The stories in this book exist in no small measure because of the devotion of these individuals. Volunteers have been the lifeblood of Children's Hospital, dating all the way back to Anna Clise, whose loss of her own child to serious illness drove her to try to prevent other families from having to live through a similar sorrow.

The devotion of Children's volunteers is not something I've just heard or read about—I've seen it firsthand. I saw it in my late wife Mary, a long time trustee and fund raiser, who was practically as committed to, and protective of, Children's Hospital as she was of her own children. And I'm proud to say that I have lived to see that tradition picked up by my son Bill and his wife Melinda, as well as my daughter, Libby.

They, too, have now become part of the living history of Children's Hospital. Sometimes, when such living histories are set down in words, they can lose their spirit. So rather than a history of all the volunteer contributions and organizations that have made the Hospital what it is today, I'd like to present that history in the language a child might use.

Those among you, dear readers, who have long been close to the Hospital might recognize the following story as containing many elements you are familiar with from your Children's Hospital journey, like the reference to the fresh air cottage—one of the precursors of the Children's Hospital we know today. That is because I have written the following as a child's version of the story of Anna Clise and all the volunteers who have given their love and lives to Children's Hospital.

Once upon a time, in a forest by the sea, there lived a woman whose name was Anna.

Anna was very, very sad. She had a son who was the light of her life. When he was sad, she was sad. When he smiled, she smiled—so much so that even the angels were jealous.

One day, the boy got very sick and Anna could not make him smile again. Alas, despite all she could do, all anyone could do, he journeyed on to heaven. The angels rejoiced to have another angel in their midst. But Anna was very, very sad.

Then one day, she was walking by the sea, and came upon an oyster. The oyster said, "Why are you so sad?" And so she told him.

"Well," said the oyster, "Within my shell I have many difficulties—irritations, you know—things that chafe and hurt and will not go away. But I have learned a secret. If you dream and if you work very hard, you can make a thing of beauty from your sadness...a pearl of great value."

And on that day, Anna declared that she would make a pearl. Her pearl would be a little house of healing for children only. Where mothers with children whose smiles had gone away could go to get their smiles back.

She called all the other mothers together and they agreed to help. They got very busy. And the men helped, too. By and by, there was a cottage on the hill where the fresh air blew; where children found their smiles again.

And often, very often, miracles happened within those walls.

Through the generations, the cottage grew on the bounty of the town. And mothers who knew the lesson of the oyster came to the cottage to make pearls of their sadness and beacons of their hope.

Of course, sometimes there were storms and the winds of change blew cruel. But if the children had a need, it rained, not cats and dogs, but pennies and dollars and all good things on the little house of healing. There was always enough—and just a little bit more—for the next stormy day that came their way.

And so it is that for generations, children have come from near and far to a place where, every day, miracles happen.

And now, dear friends, it is up to you to see that for ages and ages, henceforth and evermore, there will always be a little house of healing for children only.

For now, Anna Clise's pearl is in your hands.

For my wife Helen

*Without my precious Helen by my side these past sixty-two years,
my life could well have been devoid of real purpose.*

Thank you, Sweetheart, for everything.

Phil Smart

My experiences, my lessons learned at a Children's Hospital and Regional Medical Center in Seattle, take place every Wednesday evening and have done so for the past forty-two years. My teachers are very young, from preemie to twenty-one years old.

The lessons. . .ah, such a variety. A course in fear, a course in pain; a course in vision; a course in courage; a course in determination; a course in goal setting; a course in faith, hope, love.

Is there is a cost related to these events, these stories, which I share? No, the stories are all paid for with a little bit of time out of the third eight hours of my day—paid in full.

So in these decades, my life has been truly changed by these teachers, my "professors," as I lovingly call them.

Occasionally, there are defeats as well as victories at the miracle house. When a child loses a life struggle, the phrase we use is "See you later."

The Angels

My First Acquaintance 17

Jeff 19

Bryson 23

Tina 25

Kathy 27

Bonnie 35

Teisha 37

Darlene 39

Kitty 43

Rhonda 45

Terry 47

Colt 51

The Letter (from The Children) 55

Lynn 57

Christy 63

The Red Suit 65

Letter to God 69

Gracie 73

Dr. B 75

Kami Sutton 79

The Phone Call 83

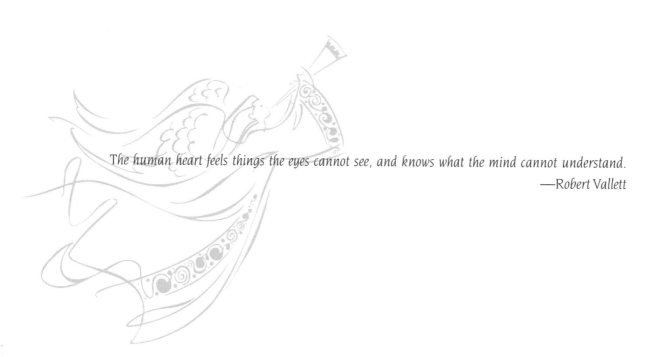

The human heart feels things the eyes cannot see, and knows what the mind cannot understand.

—Robert Vallett

My First Acquaintance

Among the hundreds and hundreds of memories that are close to my heart, I'll never forget, of course, that first night reporting for duty in One South, the teenage ward. I walked down the hall toward the nurse's station and a young RN stopped me. "Excuse me, can I be of some help?"

"Yes, my name is Phil Smart. I'm a new volunteer. I'll be here one night a week."

"What will be your responsibility?"

"I'm not sure. I asked about a manual and they said none existed, that the children would teach me."

"Well," she said, "if you'd like to meet a patient, there's a young lady down the corridor there, the first open door on the right. Why don't you go in there and make her acquaintance."

"May I ask why she's in the hospital?"

"Oh, yes, of course, she tried to commit suicide with pills."

"I beg your pardon?"

"She tried to commit suicide with pills. Go on down and make her acquaintance."

That's how it began. I appeared at the open doorway of this single-bed room and greeted that young woman.

"Hi, there."

She barely gave me a glance. "Hi. Who are you, a doctor?"

"No, I'm not a doctor."

"Are you a shrink?"

"That's a doctor."

"*Are* you a shrink?'

"No, I'm not a shrink. Do you mind if I come into your room?"

"Well, no, I guess that's okay."

And so began my first conversation with a patient in the miracle house.

I said, "Do you mind if I ask you what's going on with you in this hospital?"

She was very straightforward. "No, not at all. I tried to take my life with some pills."

"Good grief! You're about sixteen, aren't you?"

"Yes. Good guess."

"I have a daughter who's sixteen. I don't know what I would ever do if I learned she took some pills to end her life. Do you mind telling me why you did this? Must be a very good reason."

"Yes, it's a good reason. My boyfriend is in detention about sixty miles from here and he won't answer my letters and he won't talk to me on the phone. This is very, very upsetting for me to the point that I wanted to take my life."

What a memory. I know she was released but what the future brought to that young woman, I have no knowledge. No wonder that recollection is so firmly entrenched in my heart.

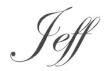

Jeff

At the beginning I started with the teenage kids because of my experience with young people in the Boy Scouts. One South was the name of the ward, and one of my first teachers was a young man by the name of Jeff. I was walking down the corridor of One South one evening, glanced in a single-bed room, and saw a strange contraption. Here this patient was upside down in a rollover-type bed. He was staring at the floor, his face not more than, I guess, two feet from the floor.

I walked in. "Hello."

He, without turning his head, said, "Hi."

"Who are you?"

"I'm Jeff. Who are you?"

"I'm a ward volunteer, Jeff. What's going on? You're upside down."

"Well," he said, "I broke my neck in a football accident. Here I am. They turn me over periodically to take the weight off my back and make sure I don't get bedsores."

I said, "I'm not comfortable speaking to you with you down there and me up here. Do you mind if I slide under your bed and we can talk a little more conveniently?"

"Why no, come on down."

So I slid under the bed. I slid under the bed in my suit and looked up and there were the most beautiful blue eyes staring down at me. I don't think our faces were more than a foot apart. Close contact, absolutely.

I was aware of footsteps coming into the room. I glanced to the left and saw a pair of white shoes. Uh-oh, an RN!

A female voice said, "What's going on down there?"

I said, "I was just talking to Jeff."

"Well, who are you?'

"I'm a ward volunteer and I know you don't know who I am but I have an idea who you are."

"Do you know that's not allowed?"

I said, "What's not allowed?"

"Well, uh, this is so unusual. I don't think you should be down there like that. Uh, are you comfortable?"

"As comfortable as I can be lying on this floor."

She said, "Well, okay." And the white shoes turned around and left the room.

And that's how the Jeff saga began. He and I became fast friends. He returned to his home in Spokane. Twenty-five years passed. Twenty-five years.

Behind a closed door in a single-bed room on Two B—rehabilitation for long-term patients—was a young man who had tried unsuccessfully to take his life with a gun.

We were chatting about his encounter with life and death. There was a bump on the closed door. I thought someone had accidentally bumped into it but it repeated, another thump. I stood up from my chair, opened the door, and there was a young man in a wheelchair wearing a blue volunteer coat, obviously a paraplegic.

He looked up at me and said, "Are you Phil?'

I said, "Yes."

"Phil Smart?"

"Yes."

"Do you know who I am?"

I looked him in the eye. "I know those eyes. I *know those eyes.*"

"I'm Jeff Sykes."

"Jeff!"

He held up his arms the best he could and placed them around my neck. He said, "It's been so long since I've seen you."

"Jeff, what are you doing here?"

He said, "I'm a ward volunteer, also. I'm trying to pay back the time that you spent with me."

The time you spent with me.

"I'm with the cancer kids up on Three, oncology and hematology. I've been doing this now for fourteen years."

"Wow! Really? Good for you. I'm proud of you."

Our relationship grew closer as the years flew by. I got to meet his dear wife, Beverly. I watched his progress at The Boeing Company, in a very responsible position. From his chair, this paraplegic is demonstrating to anyone who will listen to his story that you can take what's left of a broken life and make it count.

That's Jeff's story.

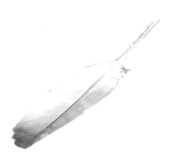

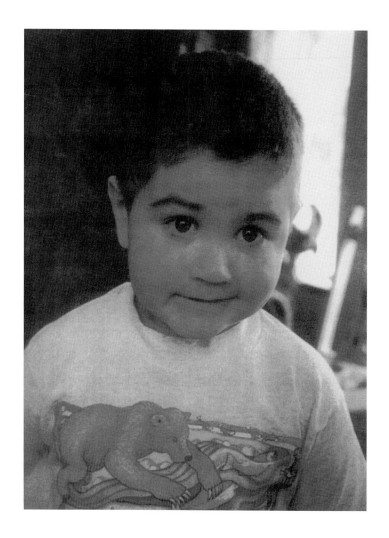

Bryson

Over the years I've learned, of course, that there is a balance at this wonderful hospital. There are pluses and there are minuses, yes. We have had some victories and we have had some defeats.

Let me tell you now about Bryson. Bryson, what a teacher! How old? Bryson's but three and a half and what a teacher he is. Is. You get the present tense. Unfortunately, Bryson was infected with a terrible virus that took away his ability to speak, his appetite, and his ability to walk. His mom rushed him over to the miracle house where he was near death's door for too long. Hope almost disappeared. Prayers came from every direction for the recovery of this dear little boy.

Well, Bryson kicked down death's door and was removed from the intensive care unit and down to rehabilitation where we became acquainted. It was a Wednesday night. Bryson was finishing his dinner. His dear mom, Susan, sat across the table from me.

I asked Susan, "Mom, I understand that this little scamp is learning to talk again. What was his first word? Do you recall what his first word was?"

And she said, "Well, Phil why don't you sing 'Old MacDonald Had a Farm' and you'll learn what his first word was."

I looked down at this beautiful young boy with the big brown eyes and started to sing as best I could, "Old MacDonald had a farm, e-i-e-i…"

"O." His first word.

"O." He's back. He's *back*.

Two weeks later, I was back at the same table and he was finishing his dinner again. I looked down at him and said, "My, you look good tonight."

Suddenly, he looked up at me and said, "Can I give you a kiss?'

His mother's eyes went as large as saucers and she mouthed the words, "He's never done this before to anyone outside the family."

I leaned closer to this young teacher and I said, "Of course, right here on this left cheek." And he raised his head. I lowered mine and he kissed me on the cheek.

I responded, "Bryson that was so nice of you. Thank you very much. May I give you a kiss now?"

He hesitated not an instant and looked up at me, his eyes widening, "Nope."

That's my teacher, Bryson.

Tina

If there was to be a title to this section of the book it might well be, "My Mission is Not Far."

Tina's thin, stockinged legs with COH, Children's Orthopedic Hospital, stitched into the white wool, hung like oversized toothpicks from the wheelchair in which she sat. They couldn't reach the floor because her normal physical growth had been inhibited by the ravages of kidney disease over the fourteen years of her life.

Big, brown, knowing eyes, tousled brown hair, and a rather reluctant smile combined with her petite size to make her a pixie-like package.

She sat quietly, intently watching the activity outside her room until greeted by my animated interruption.

"Well, hi, Tina. When did you return?"

"Oh, a couple of weeks ago, I guess. I seem to mix up the time. The hours drag so."

"And when do you get to go back home?"

"I hope by the week's end."

"Still on dialysis?"

"Yes, I'm due to be hooked up again in a few minutes."

"Just one kidney, right?"

"Yes, it's my mom's and it stopped working some months ago."

"What now?"

"Well, they want to remove it. I'll go on machine dialysis and then wait till we find a good one for me."

"How long will that take?"

"I don't know, hopefully soon. I've had so much happen to me that I can't count on anything for sure. I'll just wait."

I turned to leave, waving again at the courageous young friend in the chair. And, of course, the question in my mind begged again and again for an answer: Where can I find a kidney for Tina?

My mission is not far.

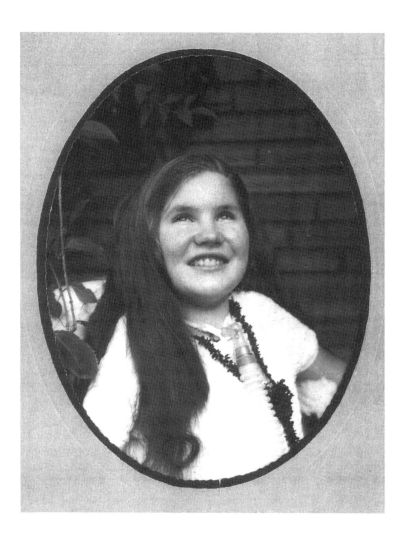

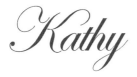

Kathy

Her name was Kathy, Kathy with a K.

At age ten, she accompanied a rifle target-shooter to a range where he was going to improve his accuracy. She stood and watched.

As he shot, the gun misfired. The bullet didn't come out the front end of the gun, the muzzle. It came out the side of the gun and struck this ten-year-old in the left side of her neck, coursed through, and cut her spinal cord in two.

In that instant, everything stopped working for that child. A trachea tube was inserted. She had no ability to move anything in her body but her head and her tongue.

Rushed to the miracle house from a faraway place, she was given every assist by the talent in that wonderful hospital.

I met her early in her rehabilitation for long-term patients. She was under a pink coverlet and didn't want to speak. The trachea tube had been inserted, but she was still getting used to it. You know, with a trachea tube, you speak with the air coming in, not like we speak with the air going out. And there she was, on a breathing machine, receiving twenty-four-hour-a-day care, and moving nothing but her head and her tongue.

We became very closely acquainted. I explained that rehabilitation accommodates the long-term patients. Kathy won first prize for long-term stay at our miracle house. She was there for ten years. I watched her grow from a frightened young ten-year-old child into a twenty-year-old lady.

She changed my life. I called her "Blue Eyes," because hers were a beautiful shade of blue. She called me "Grasshopper." I move around a lot, you see.

This young lady quickly showed her artistic talent. One Wednesday night when I arrived, someone had placed a paintbrush in her mouth and a pallet of colorful paints on the tray in front of the chair where she sat. I could hear the breathing machine, that noisy, noisy visitor.

"What are you doing?" I asked.

"I'm making a painting."

"What for?"

"I'm going to enter it in the county fair."

"Why?"

"I want to see what it will sell for."

I want to see what it will sell for.

Several weeks later, another Wednesday night, she was so excited, "Grasshopper, Grasshopper! They sold my painting."

"They what?"

"They sold my painting."

"And what did they give you?"

"They gave me a piece of paper."

"And where's the paper?"

She nodded towards it, "Over there."

I retrieved the piece of paper. It was a check. I'll never forget the date. It was August 27, 1972, thirty-one years ago.

She said, "Grasshopper, how do we turn it into money?"

"Well, you'll have to endorse it."

"Endorse? What's that?"

"Well, I'll turn this piece of paper over and I'll put a large pen in your mouth, a thick-barreled pen with a felt tip on it, and you can write your name."

I did.

She did, Kathy, with a K.

"Where's my money?"

"You really want me to cash this?"

"Yes, I do. I want my money."

I reached into my change pocket and cashed her check. On that tray in front of her, I dropped a quarter, followed by another quarter, followed by a dime. Sixty cents, that's all her painting brought at the county fair.

It really was a beautiful painting. It was called "Dad's Tree." Dad's tree, from the kitchen of her home. Dad's tree. Sixty cents. Had it been me I would have said no more, no more. All the work, all the emotion I put into this painting and it sold for sixty cents? No more.

That's not at all what she said. This young teacher looked up at me and said, "I'll do better next time."

I'll do better next time.

And did she? Of course, this bright spirit. At age sixteen she was still painting by mouth and turned out two Christmas cards. One, called "Ski Site," was small in size. It contained, and I counted them, twenty-five little green fir trees on a white background. The second was perhaps even more appropriate for the holiday season. On the front were three figures: a tall figure in front and a small figure in back separated by a donkey. Must have been Joseph and Mary headed for no room at the inn.

The hospital sold forty-five thousand of these Christmas cards. Forty-five thousand, and the proceeds went where? To the Uncompensated Care Fund, that's where she dictated the profits should go.

And you ask, "Uncompensated Care Fund, what's that?"

Since 1907, our miracle house has never turned away a family or a patient for inability to pay. This past year, they absorbed almost thirty million dollars. This was not a unique or one-

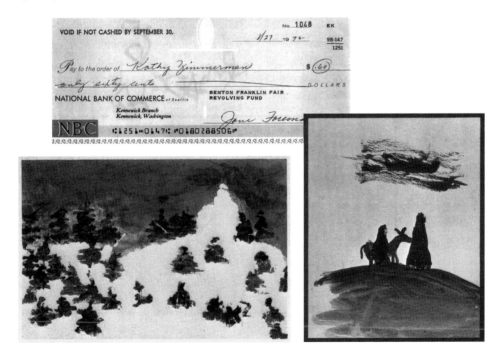

time program. The hospital has followed this pattern since its inception.

And what about Kathy with a K? She had a strong faith; she burnished my own. At age sixteen, that same year, on a Wednesday night, I looked down at her, "Blue Eyes, aren't you bitter about this experience? Aren't you bitter you've been in that bed now for four years?"

She looked back up at me and said, "Not at all. God chose me to have this experience and I would have been bitterly disappointed had he chosen anyone else."

Oh, what a teacher! God chose me. *God chose me.*

Not long after that, I again asked her a question "When are you going to get up and walk?" Are you surprised that I asked her? Well, I did.

"Oh," she said, "I'm going to get up and walk."

"Where are you going when you get up and walk?"

"Out of this bed and down that corridor out there right in front of the nurse's station. There'll be three of us."

"Three of us? Who?"

"Well, I'll be in the middle, of course. You'll be on one side and Jesus will be on the other." Such a great faith.

Kathy celebrated her sixteenth birthday in a unique way. She mouth-addressed invitations to more than twenty people. The location of the birthday celebration was at the top of the Space Needle. She had a brand new dress, long and white. What a vision.

I was concerned about choosing a special gift for this very important sixteenth birthday. I settled on a letter which I read aloud at the appropriate time at the top of the Space Needle.

To my dear young teacher:

November 22, 1975

Sweet Sixteen. What visions and feelings come to mind when these two words relate to my dear friend, Kathy.

It has been almost five years now since we first met. What changes you have brought to your life. From a bundle of fear huddled beneath the pink coverlet, you have become a beautiful, mature young lady—self-confident, self-reliant, and filled to overflowing with a vibrant spirit.

The little-girl things of yesterday have been put away: the Girl Scout Cookies, Merit

Badges, and Raggedy Ann dolls are all gone now; earrings, perfumes, lipsticks and intellectual treasures adorn your shelves.

With your artistic talents honed to a professional stature, your plans for living and working in the real world have taken on a deeper meaning.

Yet, throughout this transformation, some things haven't changed and, God willing, never will; your warm smile, the dancing lights in your lovely eyes, and the strength of your steel-strong spirit meld all of your character traits—honesty, compassion, and sensitivity, to name but a few.

All of these things are cemented together with an abiding and deep-seated faith. Throughout the years, I have found you ministering to me in ways beyond description.

May your next years yield everything your sixteen-year-old heart might wish for: peace, contentment, and finally, fulfillment of those most precious dreams of all, those you keep hidden from everyone but God.

You are precious and priceless. Happy birthday!

Love,
Grasshopper

I had many assignments during this ten-year period. I had to learn the names of all her goldfish. There must have been forty-seven of them, all her goldfish. I was in charge of trimming her Bonsai tree and one night, unfortunately, I trimmed it too short.

"Grasshopper, you've cut off too much. I'm terribly upset. Go home."

I grinned and said, "Okay, I'm going home early, but I'll be back next week."

Such a relationship.

Kathy passed away in 1980. For a long time afterward, I tried to locate her mother in Eastern Washington. Unsuccessful, I tried many, many telephone efforts. No luck. Twenty-two years passed.

Yes, it was twenty-two years and I had a phone call from the volunteer office. "Mr. Smart, there is a lady here asking if you are still a ward volunteer. I told her that, yes, you still work here. She asked how to get in touch with you, and I said we could do that. Phil, she said her name is Ina and she's Kathy's mother."

"Who?"

"Ina, Kathy's mother."

Twenty-two years and Kathy's mom was at the miracle house. What for? To see Bryson, that brown-eyed three-and-a-half-year-old.

"Ina, how long will you be here?" I asked.

"Just until tomorrow."

"May I meet you?"

The next day at noon, we threw ourselves into each other's arms in tears, remembering twenty-two years, Kathy's mom and the Grasshopper.

We sat together on Two B, right next door to where Kathy spent ten years, right across that corridor. That's where Bryson lived.

Unbelievable story? Absolutely. Coincidence? No, I think not. Part of God's plan.

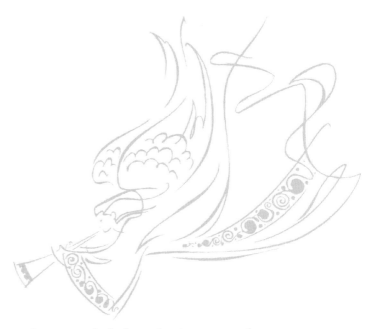

We are, each of us, angels with only one wing; and we can only fly by embracing one another.
—Luciano De Crescenzo

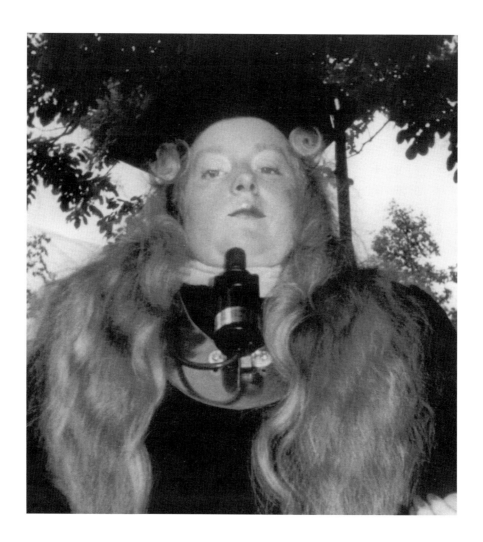

Bonnie

Bonnie, an Alaskan girl, was ten when she arrived at the miracle house.

One night, her brother was unloading a rifle and it discharged a bullet from where he sat in his bedroom. It coursed through the adjoining bedroom wall and ricocheted off Bonnie's bed where she sat next door. It struck her in the neck, bruising her spinal cord to the degree that everything stopped working in this young lady's body, with the exception of her head and her tongue.

Rushed to the miracle house by air, she was, of course, placed on a breathing machine. A trachea tube was inserted in her neck and her rehabilitation began.

We became acquainted and, by coincidence, she lived right across the corridor from Kathy with a K. You'll recall that story, Kathy with a K, who was at the hospital for ten years.

Bonnie was not destined to be there that long. After they repaired her as best they could, she flew back to Fairbanks and reentered the educational system.

She always called me Santa and kept my wife, Helen, and me informed of her progress. She would write us notes—by mouth, of course, because she couldn't move anything but her head and her tongue and remained on a respirator twenty-four hours a day, in a bed, on a gurney, in a chair with twenty-four-hour caregivers. She resumed her education, taking a bus to school with all her machinery attached.

One day, in a gray envelope addressed to Santa and Mrs. Claus, we learned of her graduation from Fairbanks High School. In a wheelchair, moving nothing but her head and tongue, she was now a high school graduate.

Four years later another invitation to Santa and Mrs. Claus announced the graduation of Bonnie Linel Barber from the University of Alaska in Fairbanks. Now she was a college graduate in a chair, on a ventilator with twenty-four-hour-a-day care.

Five years later, another letter addressed to Santa and Mrs. Claus announced the award of a master's degree in rehabilitation therapy for Bonnie Linel Barber from the University of Illinois.

She was on campus during this five-year stint, and returned, not to Fairbanks but to

Anchorage.

She applied for and received a job with Access Alaska monitoring and couseling a group of sixty-five drug addicts, alcoholics, and medically challenged people. She did this for about nine years and then retired after she had a relapse.

Our association has been wonderful for twenty-eight years. On her thirty-eighth birthday, she gave me a new assignment.

"Santa," she said, "I now want to get my doctorate."

"Your doctorate, Bonnie, are you serious?"

"Absolutely."

"In what field?"

"Clinical psychology. Now, you must find a college or university that is able to furnish me the material for this online. I can't travel anymore, obviously. And so, that's your assignment."

Now, let's put that to one side for a minute and get to Teisha.

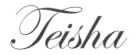

Teisha

Teisha came to Seattle from Fairbanks, Alaska, at age sixteen. Her accident occurred in a car rollover. Her neck was broken. She became a paraplegic as in contrast to Bonnie's quadriplegic condition. Teisha could move her head, was not on a breathing machine anymore, and we became acquainted. She was at the miracle house for quite an extended period of time. She, too, returned to her home in Fairbanks, after her stay in the hospital. An Athabascan Indian woman, very handsome, Teisha was bitter about her accident. Her dear mom, Marie, kept me informed of her progress through the educational system.

Recently, I received an invitation to a commencement at the University of Alaska at Fairbanks where this remarkable young lady would receive her master's degree in community psychology.

The day before the commencement there was to be a barbeque and there was a little invitation to that as well.

I presented myself at Teisha's home on the Saturday before the commencement, just in time for the barbeque, surprising Teisha and her family, especially her blessed mother.

Alaska Airlines return flight from Fairbanks to Seattle had a stopover in Anchorage, which allowed me to visit that other master's degree holder, Bonnie, in her little apartment.

Bonnie and her caregiver, Jane, invited me for dinner. Jane served me a piece of salmon, delicious, and a glass of water at bedside next to Bonnie who was also enjoying this delicacy.

After dinner, Bonnie reminisced once again about our association of twenty-eight years. She asked Jane to bring in a picture that she wanted to give to me to bring back to Seattle. It's a beautiful picture: snow-capped mountains surrounded by a full rainbow, and flying right into your eyes is a beautiful bald eagle.

Bonnie said, "If I can't walk like everyone else, I want to fly like an eagle. Do you know this eagle's name?"

"No, Bonnie, of course I don't."

"His name is Freedom."

What a story. What a story of that teacher.

I bid her aloha and told her again, as I have so many times, how proud I am of what she's done with her life, influencing others—a perfect example of courage, determination and goal-setting.

She said, "Santa, this is a very heavy load."

It was the first time she'd ever shared that point of view with me.

Two young ladies, Alaskans by birth, each with a master's degree, one a quadriplegic, the other a paraplegic. Two of my teachers. I love to tell their story.

Teisha now works and is in charge of counselors out in the villages where young, growing, Athabascan Indians receive assistance for life's emotional and physical challenges.

Darlene

Darlene, Darlene. A student at Mount Vernon High School in Washington, she and her family moved to Luxembourg, Germany, a long, long way from the miracle house.

She came to the miracle house when she was fifteen years old. As she was getting off the school bus in Luxembourg one afternoon, she was struck by a car. There was severe damage to her knees but even more importantly and more seriously, she hit her head and went into a deep coma. Flown back to Mount Vernon, she was in the hospital there for two nights and then taken to the miracle house, where we met.

She had no means to communicate. She would raise her fingers in a "V" sign and giggle unnaturally, much like a developmentally disabled child might, but that was all she did.

We were introduced, "Mr. Smart, this is Darlene. Darlene, this is Mr. Smart." There was the giggle, then the peace sign.

Each Wednesday night, they carefully removed her from bed and placed her tenderly in a banana cart—a long, narrow, coaster wagon-type vehicle with safety wheels on all sides. I proceeded, as a storyteller, to push her around the hospital while we pretended. We'd pretend we were a helicopter flying over the Grand Canyon or we'd pretend we were on the Amtrak train headed for Portland or even a Greyhound bus headed for Chicago.

A giggle and a peace sign. A giggle and a peace sign.

The professionals in the long white coats, for whom I have such high regard, said, "Phil, don't get your hopes too high. This is a very, very severe coma. The longer that she is like this, the less likely that she will ever recover."

I would talk to her and she'd giggle. And the long white coats would ask, "Why do you speak to her?"

"Well, over the years, my other teachers have taught me to read eyes and I believe she's in there. She's truly in there."

"Oh, yes," said the long white coats. "Oh, yes."

But true to the forecast, the days and weeks and months went by. Suddenly a year had gone by and we still had a giggle and a peace sign. Darlene turned sixteen.

It was a memorable night when I was saying goodnight to her roommates in the four-bed room. A young woman named Kitty was in bed four. She was a precocious seventeen-year-old who always called my by my first name. She was at the miracle house because she dove into a lake too shallow for her body and became a paraplegic. She was known for directing me. "Phil do this" and "Phil do that."

So it wasn't out of character, that particular Wednesday night at nine o'clock, for her to say, "Phil, you haven't said goodnight to bed two."

Bed two was where Darlene was living at the time. So I went over to bed two and leaned over the rail. Her eyes were closed. I thought she must be asleep. And so I said, "Good night, sweetheart, I'll see you next week." I raised my head to leave and her eyes opened and she looked up at me and said three words. What do you suppose they were?

"I love you."

After a year.

Well, I was lime jello inside. I was tears head to foot as I turned to Kitty and said, "Kitty, is this a bad trick? Has it taken you twelve months to teach her to say those three special words?"

"No, no, Phil," she responded. "Her mother came down from Mount Vernon this past Sunday. She came out of the coma completely and we saved this as a surprise for you."

Surprise, indeed.

I still thought it was a trick. Darlene's last name is Shriver. That must be German or Austrian and, if so, perhaps she understood German. Well, I know a little German myself and I began to count in German.

I looked down at those big brown eyes and said, "*Eins, zwei, drei.*"

She looked back up at me and said, "*Vier, fünf, sechs.*" Four, five, six.

She's completely out of the coma. She returned to high school, graduated, married, had two daughters and I lost track of this particularly memorable teacher.

How did I lose track? Kitty, who kept me informed, said, "See you later" at age twenty-three.

Time passed until two years ago the phone rang at the office and it was for me.

"Is this Mr. Smart?'

"Yes, it is."

"The hospital Mr. Smart?"

"Yes, it is. Who is this?"

"This is Darlene."

"Darlene. For heaven sake, where are you?"

"I'm in Seattle."

"And why did you call me?"

"I wanted to see how you are."

"Well, I'm just fine. Darlene, I don't want to embarrass you but I must ask, how old are you now?"

"I'm forty-two years old."

"Forty-two, my heavens how time flies."

"I must hang up now," she said, "but before I do, I want to tell you two things."

"And what might they be?"

"First of all, I love you, and second, you're in my prayers every single night."

The rewards of spending just a little bit of time giving of myself are rich indeed.

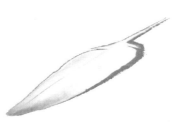

What lies behind us and what lies before us are small matters compared to what lies within us.
—Ralph Waldo Emerson

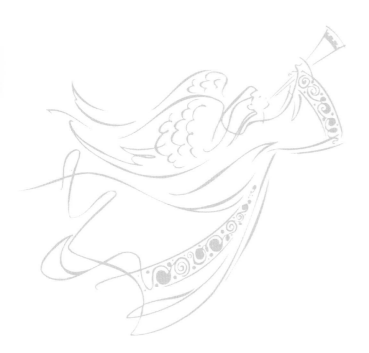

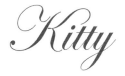Kitty

The nearby lake beckoned the neighborhood swimmers, the summer sun promising a lazy afternoon for these high school friends.

Suddenly, serenity turned to calamity. Kitty had dived into water too shallow for her body and she lay helpless on the water's surface. Eager hands moved her quickly to the shore.

More professional aid was promptly called and she soon found herself landing adjacent to the miracle house. The forty-five-minute helicopter trip was now a blur in her short-term memory.

Her injury allowed her limited ability to move her arms and shoulders, but there was no movement below her chest. She was a paraplegic who would now call her wheelchair home.

We became good friends. Attending her high school graduation, I dreamed with her of further education which would allow her life vision of teaching children to become reality.

The years passed and her dream was closer and closer to becoming true when, unexpectedly, her kidneys began to fail. Dialysis became the master of her time, dulling her enthusiasm and blunting her desire.

Once again, back in the miracle house, we spoke of the future and determined her goals. She found comfort in a wall-hung plaque on which encouraging words reminded her:

"I am the place where God shines through.
He and I are one, not two.
I will not fear, nor fret, nor plan.
My place is where and as I am.
And if I be relaxed and free
He will carry out his plan through me."

It was a special message of reality, for it had been sent to me by my mother, written by an anonymous author, when I was in North Africa during World War II.

Kitty was another great teacher, a strong Christian. Her letters to me in her early twenties always included a Bible verse reference. One of these, received in February 1977, was particularly memorable. It included a lovely snapshot of her. At first I had to look up the verse, Isaiah 40:31; now it is a favorite, committed to memory:

"Those who wait upon the will of God shall renew their strength. They shall mount up with wings as eagles. They shall run and not be weary. They shall walk and not faint."

Though no longer with us, Kitty still teaches me after all these decades. See you later, my dear, dear Kitty.

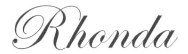

Rhonda

Comas are scary things. You don't know if, when, or how recovery might occur. And so it was with Rhonda, a fifteen-year-old from Alaska, whose accident left her unresponsive in room 207.

Her frantic mom looked for answers from anyone, finally speaking with me.

"Ma'am, I'm just a volunteer, but over the years I've seen a number of young patients with similar injuries make remarkable recoveries. As difficult as it might be, patience is the virtue most required."

Weeks passed. Some movement returned to her right side. Hearing and sight were welcomed with joy, yet speech remained a stranger. An alphabet board placed on the arms of her wheelchair became the communication device. Her fingers slowly, ever so slowly, spelled the words that surfaced in her hazy thought process.

It was another magical Wednesday night. My chat with Rhonda, certainly one-sided, brought a welcome smile of thanks to her uplifted face and she began to trace words to me on her alphabet board. The left hand worked the letters, "I L-O-V-E Y-O-U."

I have been the recipient of many comments and thank-yous over the decades, but none was quite so meaningful, memorable, and touching as this one from a heart and mind returning to reality, a healing.

It was another miracle, of course.

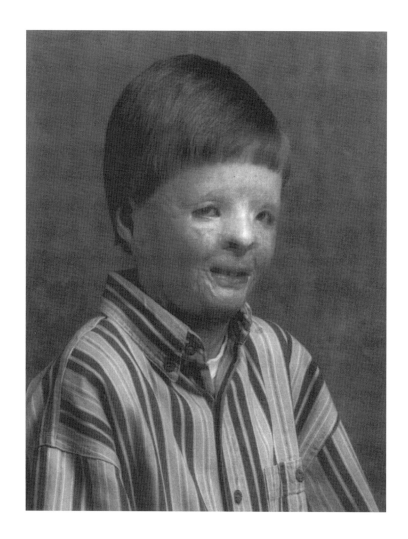

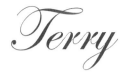
Terry

Seven-year-old Terry was a burn victim. His small body was almost consumed, head to toe, in that conflagration.

He came to the miracle house and some physician magicians restored as best they could his facial features, toes, arms, and fingers. He wore a mask and was subject to teasing almost beyond description.

He and I became good friends. We raced small model automobiles up and down the hospital corridor.

Helen and I received an invitation that winter to attend a large function—dinner in a big hotel. The Anti-Defamation League was honoring us with a plaque and they asked if I could bring a patient from the hospital. Well, who else would I choose but my young teacher, Terry?

During the program, after the entrée, it was time for me to introduce Terry. And so, I raised him up by his arms and stood him on a chair so he could see the audience and the audience could see this young man. Raising the microphone close to his lips I said, "Ladies and gentlemen, I want you to meet one of my great young teachers at the miracle house. This is young Terry.

"Terry, now that Christmas has come and gone, why don't you tell this audience what was the greatest gift you received?"

He hesitated not an instant, looked out over the crowd, and said one word, "Eyelids."

You could have heard a pin drop in that large dining hall.

"Why eyelids?" you say. Well, until he received his gift, he couldn't close his eyes and go to sleep and we would place towels over that precious face in order for him to get some rest.

Years later, I was in a large marketplace and a lady came toward me pushing a cart, looking at me. I didn't know her, didn't recognize her from anyplace that I had been before. She must have been at the dinner.

Passing me, she looked into my eyes and said one word: "Eyelids."

The lesson in this was how we take for granted so much of this life, of this world, the beauty of a sunrise or a sunset; the magnificent colors of flowers that surround us; the smell of rain;

the ability to taste, and touch, and see, and hear. We take so much for granted. Eyelids. *Eyelids.*

Is that the end of the story?

Oh, no it isn't. Time passed. I lost track of Terry. He moved from one foster family to another and then an e-mail came into the dealership: Attention Mr. Smart.

It was from Terry.

Dear Mr. Smart,

Will you please call me at this number?

And so I did. "Terry, where are you?"

"Well, I'm just a ferry ride from where you live, across the Sound, in Bremerton."

"How are you?"

"I'm fine."

"How old are you now?"

"Well, I'm fifteen."

The years had passed, all too quickly.

"Mr. Smart, can you and Mrs. Smart attend my graduation from middle school? It'll happen in just a couple of weeks. Will you come, please?"

"Certainly."

And so, Helen and I were there. We drove off the ferry and how did we recognize this young man?

We saw a hooded figure standing on the left side of the road, the hood pulled up over his head and the sleeves of the jacket too long, to cover the burned fingers. It was Terry, six-foot-two.

We followed him out to the graduation and sat through the excitement of his moving from middle school to high school.

At the conclusion of the ceremony we walked out to the car and prepared to catch the ferry boat back to Seattle. He came to me, looked down, and said, "Can I please give you a hug?"

I looked up. "Of course."

And so he gave me a hug, kissed me on the cheek, and whispered in my ear, "I love you. I love you."

As a matter of coincidence, thirty minutes ago the phone rang. It was Terry informing me that he would have another operation this summer on his left arm; operation, after operation, after operation.

"What did he teach you?" you ask.

Oh my—courage, determination, life-planning, how to handle pain.

What a teacher. What a teacher.

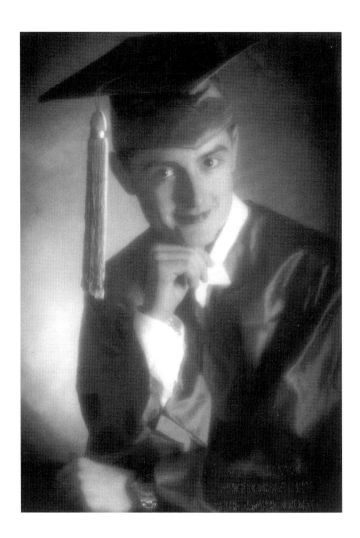

Colt

Colt and I met about the time that cancer arrived in his right leg. What a young man, age ten at the time. Our relationship lasted for the better part of seven years until we finally said to each other, "See you later."

Those years in between were filled with events that cried for a story to be told.

The son of a single-parent mom, a blessed woman by the name of Patty, Colt had two older sisters. During this event, those three were so supportive of Colt in the wins and losses of his life.

He called me "Max" for Maxwell Smart, that television actor of years gone by. "Max this" and "Max that," that was our relationship. Through this period of treatment at the miracle house, he endured probably fifteen, sixteen, seventeen procedures. He generally would call me the day before.

"Max?"

"Hi, Colt, how's it going?"

"Well, I'm going in again tomorrow."

"Really."

"Yes."

"What time?"

"Ten o'clock. Will you be there?"

"Yes, I'll be there."

And I had the pleasure, so many times, of lifting him up onto the gurney just before they wheeled him into the operating room, kissing him on the forehead, telling him, "Thank you, Colt, for being such a great teacher. You've shown me courage that I was not aware of, determination, and you've shared our friendship. Thank you."

He would respond quickly, "I'll be out of recovery in about three hours. Will you be there?"

"Yes. I'll be there."

I was there the night when the surgeon came in and gave Colt the news. "Colt the cancer is back in your leg and we're going to have to amputate it above the knee."

"What did you say?"

"The cancer is back, Colt, and we're going to have to amputate your leg above the knee."

As was typical of this young teacher of mine, he replied quickly, "Let's get on with it."

And so, the amputation was made and his leg healed. Patty and I were in the room when his prosthesis, this stranger, was attached to the stump of his right leg. We were both in tears as this young hero of ours took his first step.

"Colt, are you going to call this thing something?"

He said, "Yes," and with that sly grin he turned his head and said, "I'm going to call it Max."

Each time he took a step with that new leg, I was there.

Patty's call came mid-day two years ago, May 3. "Max, you had best come. Colt needs to see you."

Almost graduated from high school, this young man was now facing reality. I walked up the stairs to his room. He was in the reclining chair. Jesse, his loveable labrador, had his nose in his lap. Colt was on oxygen. Could hear but couldn't speak. I was able to speak with him for an hour and a quarter, holding his right hand. Another memory.

Patty called again the next day. "Max, Colt passed away this morning at 6:30." I revisited his home and sat in the living room sharing a second day with the family.

So many of his schoolmates, seniors in high school, came through the front door, walked up those steps, and said, "See you later," to their dear friend.

The memorial service was also memorable: four eulogies and five of his male friends had "Colt" tattooed on their left shoulder, attesting to their relationship with Colt, the teacher.

During those treatment years, Colt had said to his mother on a number of occasions, "Mom, if I can't walk like everyone else, I want to fly like an eagle."

"What?"

"I want to fly like an eagle."

That was not forgotten as the urn was picked out for the ashes of my dear friend, Colt.

I had the pleasure and honor of driving him home from the mortuary. We talked again on that all-too-short trip.

His urn? An eagle.

He rests in the living room of that loving family's home: Colt, the eagle.

Five weeks after the service, a phone call again came from Patty. She said, "Max, something strange is happening."

"What's that?"

"Well, in our summer home, I'm beginning to find feathers in the yard. What do you make of that?"

"Oh, Patty, that's a slam dunk. Colt has on his eagle wings and is checking up on mom."

"You really think so?"

"I'm positive."

It wasn't but days later that I opened the locked front door of the dealership at 8:00 a.m. My eyes were startled to see on the carpet a feather—an eagle feather, black and white with mottled grays. Colt, my dear friend, checking up on Max.

A few days later, Patty called yet again. "Max, guess what? I'm beginning to find white feathers now."

"Come on, Patty, you're teasing."

"No, I'm finding white feathers."

"He must have on his angel wings, Patty. Double duty, checking up on his blessed mom."

Days later, I began to find white feathers in the strangest places, inside the automobile, on the roof of a car, in the gateway to our home.

White feathers. My dear young teacher making certain that I knew he was back, checking up on me, confirming that everyone has a guardian angel, and that I should tell the story to prove that fact.

Colt, what a teacher. What a mother. What a family. Colt.

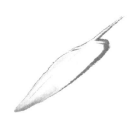

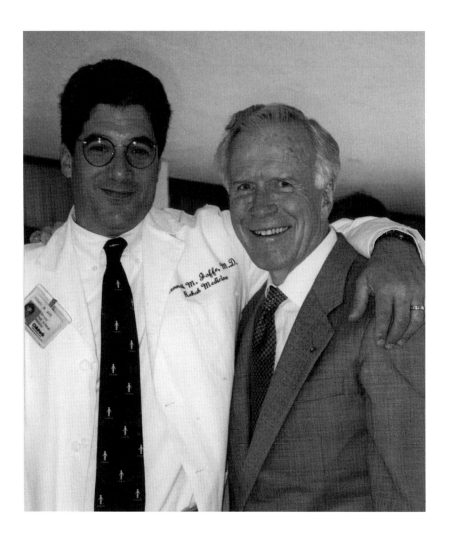

The Letter

This letter was recently discovered:

CHRISTMAS

Dear Doctor,

Some of us can't speak yet. Some of us can't speak clearly and some of us can't speak at all so we're writing this.

We understand Santa is calling on you so we sent it to the North Pole to make certain you'd have this before Christmas.

You're always so busy that we never seem to see you as we leave the hospital after you've said we're well enough to go home.

Oh, yes, we see you flying around everywhere in your white coat but there are so many people around we'd be embarrassed to talk to you then. We've seen you in the operating rooms, the recovery rooms, in casting, the lab, outpatient, in rehabilitation therapy and physical therapy, in ICU and ACU, the cafeteria, and the board room and administration.

We guess you go to all these places as part of your busy job but we seem to see you at the oddest hours, too, very late at night, early in the mornings. Don't you ever sleep?

You've placed your cool hands on our hot foreheads and stood by our bedsides for hours pondering what's best for us. You've sat for hours in meetings planning for our futures, both in the hospital and after we leave it. You've talked to our parents and our brothers and sisters about us and encouraged them when they were blue.

Right now, we'd like to thank you for being our friend and treating each of us as if we were one of your own family.

Well, we probably should stop now. If we don't get this in the mail soon, Santa is sure to miss the delivery to you.

We could sign this with many names you'd know, like Darlene, Robert, Kitty, Jason, Gracie, Terry, Kathy, Matthew, Rosa, Beth, Cher, Tammy, and hundreds of others but perhaps it is best just to say thank you, and we love you,

The Children

Love

If I had the gift of being able to speak in other languages without learning them, and could speak in every language there is in all of heaven and earth, but didn't love others, I would only be making noise. If I had the gift of prophecy and knew all about what is going to happen in the future, knew everything about everything, but didn't love others, what good would it do? Even if I had the gift of faith so that I could speak to a mountain and make it move, I would still be worth nothing without love. If I gave everything I have to the poor people, and if I were burned alive for preaching the Gospel but didn't love others, it would be of no value whatever. Love is very patient and kind, never jealous or envious, never boastful or proud, never haughty or selfish or rude. Love does not demand its own way. It is not irritable or touchy. It does not hold grudges and will hardly even notice when others do it wrong. It is never glad about injustice but rejoices whenever truth wins out. If you love someone you will be loyal to him no matter what the cost. You will always believe in him, always expect the best of him, and always stand your ground in defending him. All special gifts and powers from God will someday come to an end, but love goes on forever. Someday prophecy, and speaking in unknown languages and special knowledge — these gifts will disappear. Now we know so little, even with our special gifts, and the preaching of those most gifted is still so poor. But when we have been made perfect and complete, then the need for these inadequate special gifts will come to an end, and they will disappear. It's like this: when I was a child I spoke and thought and reasoned as a child does. But when I became a man my thoughts grew far beyond those of my childhood, and now I have put away the childish things. In the same way, we can see and understand only a little about God now, as if we're peering at His reflection in a poor mirror; but someday we are going to see Him in His completeness, face to face. Now all that I know is hazy and blurred, but I will see everything clearly, just as God sees into my heart right now. There are three things that remain — faith, hope, and love — and the greatest of these is love.

1 Corinthians 13

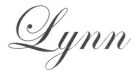

Lynn

Another Wednesday evening, this one in October. I was midway through the storytelling, playing checkers with those in the wheelchairs, guiding the children in the rehabilitation unit, when a nurse's aide approached me. "I've become acquainted with a young lady up on Three A whom I believe you should meet."

"What's her name and why is she a patient here?"

"Her name is Lynn. She's fifteen years old and has cystic fibrosis."

I walked away from Two B and up the nearby stairs. I quickly reflected on CF, that insidious disease of the lungs—thick mucus causing labored breathing, frequent hospital checkups, state-of-the-art new prescription applications, and all-too-clear and accurate forecasts of abbreviated life expectancies.

When I got to Lynn's room, introductions were quickly shared, first with her mom, then with the dark-eyed brunette sitting upright in her bed, who wasted not a moment in asking a question.

"They tell me, Mr. Smart, that I am going to live only until February, just three months away. Do you believe them?"

Over the years of my volunteering, I had learned that when challenged by an unexpected question, the first and best response was to answer by posing the question back to the asker.

"Do *you* believe them?" I asked her.

"No, of course not. What do you think?"

"Well, we've just met, but from that determined reply, I'm inclined to believe you."

What followed was that first fascinating hour when I learned about her: how she misssed so much of school being in and out of the miracle house, enduring the clinical treatments that made graduation seem but a dream; that among her likes were her dog, art, and Neil Diamond, whose tapes and records she played by the hour during her homebound days. Her faith was substantial and as time passed she burnished my own.

During that time, we together planned goals and painted life visions. I listened intently to her animated reactions as she was awarded a GED from her high school and expanded her Neil

Diamond collection due to my scouring Seattle for missing musical treasures. Lynn and her mom shared several luncheons with Helen and me, where we shared our dreams for the future. Lynn and I looked for a secret code, a passage from the Bible, which we could subtly exchange by voice and written notes.

We were encouraged by Lynn's progress, and that fated February came and went. One night, Lynn asked another question, "Do you know that Neil Diamond is going to have a concert in Texas?"

"No. You already know that I'm not nearly as current about your friends as you are."

"I wish I could see him."

I turned to the Rotary Club Wishing Well and, to her delight, arrangements were made for Lynn and her mom to fly to Dallas. The Rotarians arranged to meet them and handle everything, including tickets for concert seats close to the stage. Lynn was beside herself with excitement as she departed.

Upon her return, Helen and I waited patiently for her at the gate, her wheelchair the last to leave the aircraft.

Totally exhausted, wan, and sad, she related in soft tones the concert details. "The concert was overwhelming. He sang beautifully and the Rotarians arranged for a backstage visit with the man himself. I sat just outside his dressing room door. . .that close."

She was certain that someone miscommunicated, for word came back to her disappointed ears, "Sorry, Mr. Diamond cannot see you. His schedule is such that none of his many admirers are allowed beyond this point."

Lynn always said that had he known it was her, all the way from Seattle, that girl in the chair would have had her dream come true. She forgave him.

It was a Maui kind of day; the beauty of a glorious sunrise, rising from behind the foreboding mass of Haleakala, had forecast another twelve hours of lazy time in paradise. The golf game had been relatively easy on the morning scores. Lunch was now finished but the solitude was shattered by a nosy phone ring. "Sir, this is security. You have two visitors on their way to your condo."

Not expecting anyone, I replaced the receiver and hurried through the front door and looked up the walkway. There she was: Lynn, with her mom close by.

"Lynn, for heaven sake, what are you doing here? How did you manage oxygen bottles on the airplane? How did you make the transfer in Honolulu?" The questions tumbled out of an astonished voice box.

Her reply came from her heart. "I wanted to see you."

They must have signed releases beyond count to allow this fragile cargo to even embark on the seven-hour trip.

What followed then were five days of sightseeing, talks of her future, and the continuing Bible search for that special phrase unique to the two of us.

To the surprise of no one, she and her mom made that trip one more time, this one planned. The travel personnel were now better prepared to accommodate Lynn on her return to her beloved Maui.

A year and a half after her initial visit, two new goals were planned: learn to play golf and obtain a driver's license. The quest for the license was rather terrifying according to her mom; the drivers in her county were soon aware of this loose automotive cannon, yet all survived.

At last we found a hit on the Bible verse—the Bible story that tied our notes and chats and calls together. It was in the Book of Mark.

A synagogue official, Jarius, was blessed with a twelve-year-old daughter who became deathly sick. He sought the immediate help of Jesus, who was nearby engaged in conversation with a number of believers. "Come Master, save my daughter. She is sick unto death."

His neighbors interrupted. "Don't bother the Master, your daughter has died."

Jesus turned to Jarius and said, "Do not fear. Only believe."

Those five words became a lifeline between the two of us, sprinkled through phone calls, notes, and eye-to-eye hellos and goodbyes.

One of Lynn's greatest friends was seventeen-year-old Christy, with whom she shared a deep-seated faith and the insidious cystic fibrosis. More than once, I saw them walk down the halls of the miracle house together, animatedly exchanging giggles, holding hands, and affirming their special relationship.

During these days, Lynn's condition worsened. The checkup periods extended into weeks as newer and more exotic medicines were hopefully administered but without notable success.

Lynn's mom had shared her growing concerns and I visited this courageous teacher more frequently. It was June 25, two days before her seventeenth birthday, a down day, and to cheer her up, I composed a four-verse sonnet and affixed it to a nearby door so she could read it again and again at her leisure.

LMM, *Lynn Michelle Martin*

It has been said and proven true,
There is but one and only you
Who's graced the lives of all you've met
And reached each goal that you have set.
Your talents many, you have shared, drawing, painting.
They've been paired with smiles many.
Laughter ringing, hearts you've touched, spirits singing.
Because of you the world is brighter,
Faces smiling, burdens lighter.
And so it seems it should be written,
"It's Lynn Michelle with whom we're smitten."
And now, to you this bright June day,
We pause a moment just to say,
"We love you greatly and say again,
Thank you, charmer, for being our friend."

25 June 1987, *The Anonymous Poet*

As I left the room that morning, I looked at her damp hair, matted across her forehead, her face pale from the medicine, and asked, "How's your head?"
"Fine."
"How's your heart?"
"Fine."
"Mark 5:36, 'Do not fear. Only believe.'"
The insistent ring at 1:30 a.m. was her mom. "Lynn passed away moments ago."

"We'll be right out."

Tears blurred my vision in the accelerated fifteen-minute drive to the miracle house. Quickly up to Two A, room 207. She lay peacefully in the bed and, after asking her mom, I kissed Lynn's right cheek and murmured, "See you later."

I was asked to eulogize my teacher and I did, honored in so doing. The sonnet now sounded incomplete and so I added two more verses for her mom's memory box.

At last you're free to dance and sing.
We have no doubt that heaven will ring
Its song of joy, thanks, and laughter.
She's here at last, forever after.
And we'll recall a different us.
'Twas oh so subtle without a fuss
Who marked our lives, how changed we are,
That precious girl, who's now a star.

26 June 1987

In the memoriam card for those attending were five words: "Do not fear. Only believe."

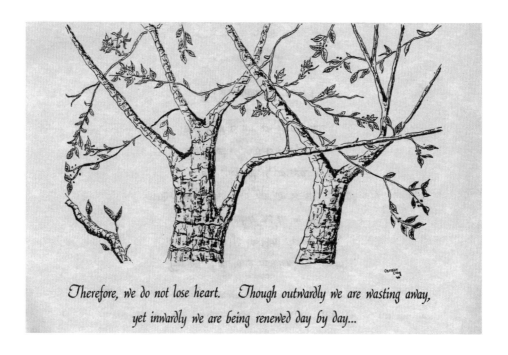

Therefore, we do not lose heart.   Though outwardly we are wasting away,
yet inwardly we are being renewed day by day...

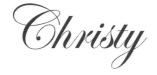

Christy

Christy, who was stronger than Lynn, was awaiting a heart-lung transplant and soon was moved from the miracle house to the University of Washington Hospital. She had to be within three air-hours of the Stanford Hospital where the transplant would be performed, the magic of a heart-lung transplant.

I had enjoyed two visits with this charming young lady and I looked forward to this Saturday morning exchange. I entered the single-bed room, quickly disappointed that she was sleeping. I left.

Monday morning, at the beginning of another busy work week, a call interrupted me. "You have a gentleman on line two."

"This is Christy's father. Were you at the hospital on Saturday?"

"Yes, mid-morning, but we didn't get a chance to visit. She was sleeping and I didn't want to disturb her, knowing how weak she has been in recent days."

"That's a real shame. She passed away yesterday morning."

This sad exchange quickly ended and I, tears again loosed, ran upstairs to a Bible sitting on the shelf.

You might guess that when I opened it at random, it was Mark 5:36, but it wasn't. No, it opened next door to the Book of Luke. Luke 8:50 read, "Do not fear. Only continue to pray and your daughter will be made well."

It was the same story, Jesus responding to Jarius, that frantic father of a sick little girl. Was it God speaking to me through the Bible pages, offering encouragement, guidance, and teaching? Of course.

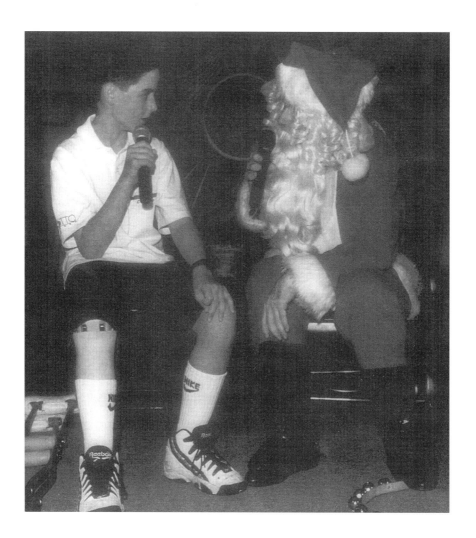

The Red Suit

Hanging in a wired enclosure for most of the year, it silently awaited a single, magical day when it would again be put to use.

The shiny black boots and large, round sleigh bells quietly rested within the cardboard box. Slowly removed from their musty storage on this special day, the items were transported to a huge building on a faraway hill.

Soon, a thin man in a blue business suit would once again be transformed into a legend as he had every year for more than a quarter of a century. First, a dusting of chalk on eyebrows and lashes to emphasize age; rouge to bring the color of the northern frost to his forehead, cheeks and nose; then the binding of pillows around the middle to affirm the familiar, plump profile. The trousers and jacket trimmed in white carried the wide, black belt much like a comfortable equator. The soft, flowing beard was affixed by bands around tender ears. With his wig carefully adjusted and his cap now in place at a jaunty angle, the transformation was complete.

Stepping into the imposing hospital lobby, sleigh bells foretelling his entrance, the annual journey began and the visit would conclude nearly six hours later.

There were 127 stops to make this day, sharing smiles and tears, belief and disbelief.

Red Suit moved from one room to another, each one different and yet, somehow, the same. Cares and hurts were forgotten as each child eagerly awaited a magical moment, a large hug, and a small Christmas package.

The hospital walls seemed to disappear momentarily before reality returned and they again became an unwelcome presence.

"He's critical with leukemia so don't linger too long," whispered the night nurse as they rounded the corner into the next room.

The eight-year-old child quietly shared his own conviction with Red Suit. "You know, what you have to have is good health, do as well as you can, and everything will turn out all right."

The child's mom leaned into the soft, white curls, seeking the comfort of a tender hug. He murmured some private words of reassurance, slowly walked to the door, and offered a farewell wave.

A young mother met him outside of the next room. "She's not able to speak, though she's seven."

A beautiful child with blond hair, blue eyes, and a warm, understanding smile awaited his entrance. Their heart strings entwined and they savored their brief exchange. The conversation was one-sided, yet her eyes spoke clearly and lovingly.

At that moment, there came an interruption. An aid from the third floor appeared in the doorway and announced, "Megan, upstairs, doesn't believe in you."

In haste, he climbed the stairs to greet her. She was involved in a coloring project.

"Hi, Megan. I'm Santa Claus."

The beautifully freckled eight-year-old looked up from her artwork, "I don't believe in Christmas. I have Hanukkah."

Her father leaned over to Santa and said, "Shalom."

Santa replied, "Ah, Shalom to you my friend. I know of the eight lights and the eternal tapers."

Turning to the next bed, Santa smiled to himself, recalling his warm relationship with a senior rabbi up the street.

"Are you her mom?" he asked the woman sitting there.

"Yes, she's mine. Eighteen years old, with cystic fibrosis, and doing as well as we can expect."

He moved closer to the bedside, bent over the still figure entwined in tubes connected to machinery, and quietly spoke a word of faith. Recalling many answered prayers, he made his way to the next room.

A tender eight-year-old heart was mending. The vivid vertical line down his chest was mute testimony to the surgical expertise performed nearly forty-eight hours earlier.

"He's doing fine!" his mother exclaimed.

His infectious grin confirmed his mother's enthusiastic remark.

And so it went, hour after hour, a sharing of joys and sorrows, hopes and fears with Red

Suit, a mysterious man who was unbelievable, yet believable since, there he was.

As forecast and heralded, it was a single day when all was meant to be right with the world, from fragile one-and-a-half pound premature babies to high-spirited young adults. Some were newly adjusting to their confining circumstances, others were veterans of long-term care, yet all were wanting, hoping, and praying for the same things: pain relief, courage, understanding, reconciliation and recovery.

The Legend heard it all, sensing the unspoken. At visit's end, he slowly removed the vestiges of the day and carefully put them away until another year would pass. Certainly, the teardrops on the red suit would have dried by then.

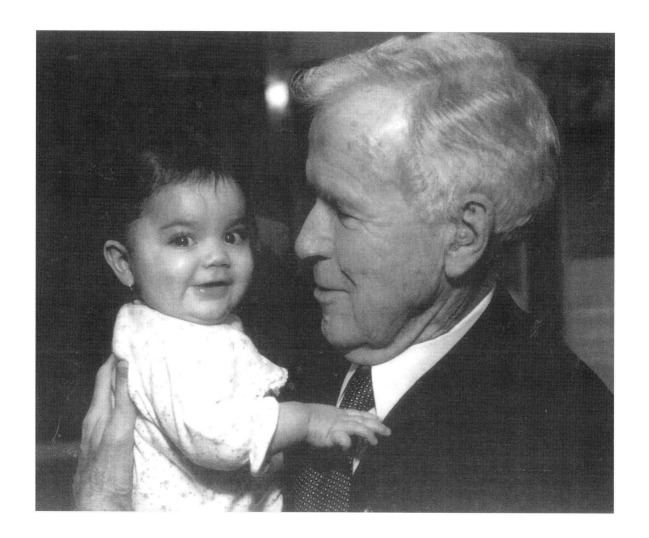

Letter to God

This letter was sent to God by me, a man who wears a red suit one day a year. I was sitting on the beach on a beautiful Maui day.

Maui, Hawaii April 29, 1986
Dear God,

In all these years I don't recall ever having written you directly before. Generally, my sentiments, wishes, hopes, and prayers have been voiced.

Certain that you receive a zillion messages, I'm not at all sure that this message will reach your eyes. But even if it doesn't, I have an abiding, deep-seated feeling that you will understand this missive, someway, somehow.

My name is Claus, first initial S, the guy in the red suit and snow-white beard who is especially apparent during the month of December each year.

Young children expect great things from me; toys, all kinds, are tops on lists of hopes. They ask Santa for trikes and skates, dolls and games, skis, puppies, diamonds for the bigger kids, and sometimes happiness and peace of mind.

Well, I'm over here in the middle of the Pacific Ocean on a little R and R. That's rest and relaxation, or recreation, as the case might be, from the rigors of calling on all the children of the world just four short months ago.

Not one to be too different from all those young people who send me their lists, I have a most special message I'd like you to hear, or read.

I'd like to tell you about a very special person I've met in my travels who, in my humble judgment, is very deserving of your special attention. This young lady's name is Lynn and she resides just outside Snohomish in the State of Washington, a part of North America.

You've probably already heard of her because I am aware that many of her acquaintances have talked to you about this most charming, almost sixteen year old. I'd like to share some of my own observations of and about Lynn, to fill in any blank spaces, so to speak.

First of all, I guess I'd have to mention her smile. One of those will blow your socks off, if I may be so bold.

Her problem, if we can call it that, is that she doesn't have the strongest lungs in the world and, as a consequence, is often challenged by not having enough air to handle her needs. This has been going on now for about six years and, while she has had excellent assistance and direction, from Children's Hospital, that's the miracle house in Seattle, in my opinion it is now necessary for a higher authority to intervene on her behalf.

Her current medication seems to be relieving some of her difficulty and all of us are hoping that this improvement will continue. Certainly there must be even more effective stuff out there that can make it easier for her and I seek that assistance now.

You see, she will celebrate her sixteenth birthday on June 27th and since that will be a most strenuous event she will have to be at peak strength by that date.

You want to know more about her? Well, she looks lovely in pink and although she refers to herself as a "pants person," she's a knockout in a skirt and blouse.

Her giggle is infectious. Her smile would melt one of my North Pole igloos and her artistic talent knows no bounds.

She's a most determined young lady, knows what she wants and where she's going. A fighter, she ignores the physical challenges she faces, yet is blessed with a vision of accomplishment for her life that is impressive and, in her judgment, perfectly obtainable.

Where do you come in, you say?

Well, I, along with millions of others, have read, and continue to read, that fascinating book about your son, his trials and tribulations, and the many observations he made during his earthly stay about what is possible if you really believe his word.

He said, "All things are possible with God." He said, "If you have faith, you can move mountains." He said, "Let go and let God."

Well, I believe this. My dear, dear friend, Lynn, believes this. Her loving, supporting family believes this and, I guess you already know, we believe this together.

So, what's the reason for this lengthy note, you say?

Simply this: I just wanted you to thoroughly understand that this is a most special life we're talking about. She has years of sharing, caring, love yet to give, talent to demonstrate, and a story to tell. A loving, knowing master like yourself, busy with all the cares in the world, could make a humble earthly family so grateful if you would reach out and touch yet another life with healing grace.

Thank you for listening, as you always do, and for reading this through.

Love, your obedient servant,
S. Claus

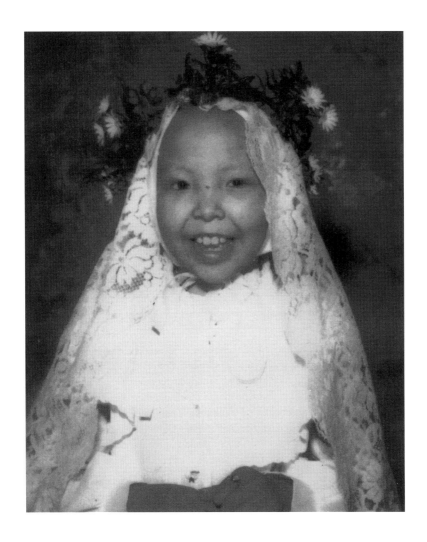

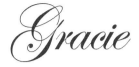 Gracie

It was one of the early stops that Christmas day. On One North, the nurse warned Red Suit that she believed this eight-year-old girl was in no mood for visitors, having given her left leg to cancer the day before.

On impulse, he entered the room with huge Jack and Jill dolls tucked under each arm. She smiled, one of those heartwarming smiles so prevalent in her Eskimo village far to the north. That began a relationship with Gracie and her parents Marie and Roy that lasted many years. Gracie moved through the Arctic school system, her balance now regained, courtesy of a carefully fitted prosthesis.

Time passed and communications exchanged at Christmastime gave witness to Gracie's growing-up years. The last letter from her mom described her daughter's unfortunate involvement in the college drug scene. Gracie took her life in her twenty-fifth year.

Her mom, now alone, gives of herself in the village. She is a friend and encourager to those facing the unexpected and unplanned events of life's challenges.

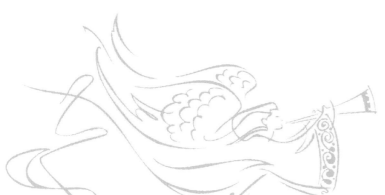

The human heart feels things the eyes cannot see, and knows what the mind cannot understand.

—Robert Vallett

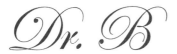 Dr. B

I called him Dr. B. Doctor. He was only ten, but wise beyond his years. I never saw him stand up. He was such a little guy. He was always in a bed, on a gurney, or in a chair.

It was October when we first met. I'll never forget the fall of that year, now decades past. He loved to be read to, each Wednesday night, and he was very attentive. I remember particularly one Wednesday evening as I appeared in the open door of his single-bed room, he lay there, surrounded by machinery making all kinds of clicks and clacks, hooked up to tubes and good paraphernalia.

Aware of my arrival, he turned his head and said, "Here comes that angel from heaven."

Here comes that angel from heaven. Me, a car dealer? Angel from heaven? I had to swallow my laughter.

Well, one particular night, I read and read and read to him. It was close to nine o'clock. He had closed his eyes, I presumed, to enter slumber-land. I slowly closed the book and put it alongside the table near his bed then rose to leave.

He quickly opened his eyes and said, "Where are you going?"

"It's almost nine o'clock and I must leave."

"Why?"

"Well, my dear friend, Dr. B, you know that at five minutes after nine I turn into a frog and you don't want to see that, do you?"

"No, no, no. When will you be back?"

"Next week. See you then."

Those next two or three months passed quickly and we found ourselves on Christmas Day. Red Suit entered Dr. B's room, now a four-bed room. He was sitting in a chair, talking on the telephone. It was obvious he was talking to his grandpa. Suddenly he said, "Grandpa, I want you to speak to the real Santa Claus." He handed me the phone.

You know that when you are in the red suit and you're on the phone, people can't interrupt you so you can be very forward and forthright in the conversation, even with a stranger, even with Dr. B's grandpa.

"Good morning, Gramps, how are ya?"

"I'm fine. How's my grandson?"

"He's fine."

"Are you sure?"

"I'm right alongside his chair here. He's doing just great. By the way, Grandpa, from where is this call coming?"

And he responded very quickly, "Aberdeen."

Aha, Aberdeen!

To those of you who don't know, Aberdeen is in the southwest corner of our beautiful state of Washington, known for lumber and fishing interests. Not too far from the miracle house, incidentally, probably two hours driving time. And so the conversation proceeded.

"Gramps, I don't understand why you're not up here at the hospital at the side of your beloved grandson, Dr. B. Look out the window. There's no snow in Aberdeen or in Chehalis or in any of the cities that my reindeer and I passed over. In fact, we had some difficulty landing the sleigh on the roof of this miracle house. There's no snow, no snow at all. So why aren't you here? I'll be just that nosey," I said, kind of apologetically, but not really. "Why aren't you here?"

His response staggered me.

"Aberdeen, Scotland."

Oh, dear! Aberdeen, Scotland, is about, I don't know, thousands of miles away. Certainly, Red Suit was not going to pick up that telephone tab and so the conversation ended rapidly.

Time passed in conversation between Dr. B and me that Christmas morning.

Suddenly, Dr. B looked up at me from the chair and said, "Santa, what do you do with pain?"

Sometimes when you're caught up in a tough question, you ask for the question to be repeated. It gives you time to figure out how you might respond.

"I beg your pardon?"

"Santa, what do you do with pain?"

"Well, look at Santa's knuckles here, all swollen and crooked; he can't even point straight to the North Pole where he lives anymore. What do *you* do with pain, my young friend?"

"Well," he responded quickly, "I take pain and put it in a box, my box of pain, and when it's filled, I wrap it in bright tissue paper and colorful ribbons and throw it away."

"Dr. B, why can't you show your pain?"

His response was immediate, as he gazed deeply into my eyes. "I can't show pain because it hurts my mother's heart."

A prescription for pain from my young friend, Dr. B.

A phone call came, one morning soon after. "Red Suit, you'd best come out to the hospital. Dr. B is slipping away."

I arrived at the miracle house just moments before he said, "See you later."

The attending staff was gathered around his room while his dear mother hovered over this young man.

I apologized for being delayed and then excused my interruption of the quietness in that room. I leaned over his still body and thanked him for being such a great teacher. Dr. B taught me about life and he taught me about death.

And now I can tell the rest of the story. He lies in a churchyard cemetery in Aberdeen, Scotland.

One of my dear RN nurse friends subsequently sent me such a kind note.

Dear Mr. Smart,

I was so moved when you spoke with Dr. B on his deathbed. We all sat in the darkness, sad with our helplessness in not being able to save Dr. B's life.

The family and several staff members encircled his bed in silence until you said, "Please forgive me while I talk with my teacher here."

You walked closer to Dr. B and I will never forget the way you spoke to him.

"My dear young friend, I'm not sure I told you often enough how much you taught me. You have been one of my finest teachers. You handled pain and fear so well. I love you and I will miss you greatly." And then you kissed him goodbye on the forehead.

When you walk into a room to spend time with a child who is attached to monitors and tubes, you see a child, not a patient. You always laugh and play with the children.

It is so profound to me because you always remind me who it is laying in that bed or sitting in that wheelchair.

I know you dress up every Christmas to play Santa but you can't fool me. I know who you are. You are Santa, who dresses up to play Phil Smart and pretends to sell cars.

Much Love,
Kathy Salmonson, Third Floor Nurse

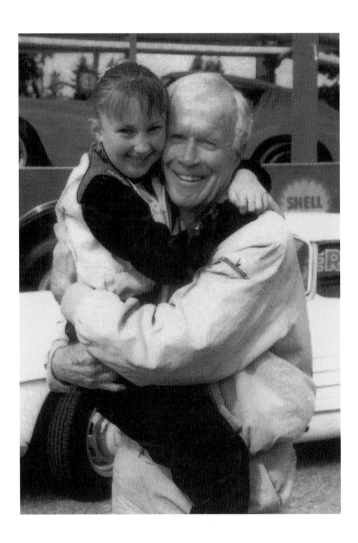

Letter from Kami Sutton

July 2, 2003

Dear Phil,

Hi, it's me, Kami Sutton. I was just thinking about you and thought I would write you a letter. I was remembering all of the good times we have had over the last six or seven years.

First of all, I want to thank you for showing me just how much of a blessing Children's Hospital really is. Even though I knew what a special place it was before I met you, you helped to open my eyes to the "triumphs and tribulations" of the "miracle house."

While reminiscing about some of our times together, I can remember the day I met you. Unlike some of your other "professors," I met you while I was outside of the hospital walls. When we first met we were at the Pacific Northwest Historics Vintage Races at Seattle International Raceway. It was the first time I had ever been to the races and I remember Don Kitch introducing me to you. I think it was love at first sight! The very next year, at the same event, we shared our first dance together, at the Saturday night barbeque. To this day, we share a dance at the Saturday night barbeque during the Historics Race Weekend, and I really look forward to it.

From there we saw each other at several other events we both attended to help Children's Hospital. I can remember at the Kick-Off Luncheon for the Children's Hospital Telethon, I was in the lobby of the Convention Center being introduced to Olympic Gymnast Kerri Strug and all of the sudden, I heard this whistle. I looked across the lobby and there you were, down on one knee with your arms extended out towards me. I remember running across the lobby and into your arms. This started a tradition for us—every time we see each other, you get down on one knee to give me a hug.

The first time I saw you, I was a patient at Children's having my twelve-hour cardiac ablation surgery. My surgery was on a Tuesday and I remember you and Jorge came to visit me on Wednesday night and brought me a Tickle Me Elmo, which I still treasure today. Having you come and visit was so special to me; it puts a smile on my face and in my heart every time I see you.

Not only do you and I share the love of racing and Children's Hospital, we also share something else that no one else can ever take away, that is our love for each other and our BIRTHDAY. I think it is so cool that we have the same birth date, September 21.

We have a very special connection in so many ways, but the friendship and love we share is by far the thing that means so much to me. I am so glad I get to see you not only while I am in the hospital as a patient, but I get to see you more while I am out of the hospital, which means I am staying healthy.

I can't wait until the Historics Weekend because I will get to spend the entire weekend with you. Thanks again for all you have done for me and for all the kids at the hospital. I love you.

Kami Sutton

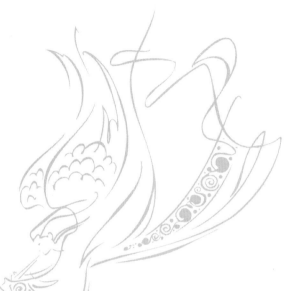

To the world you might be one person, but to one person you might be the world
                                                                    —Unknown

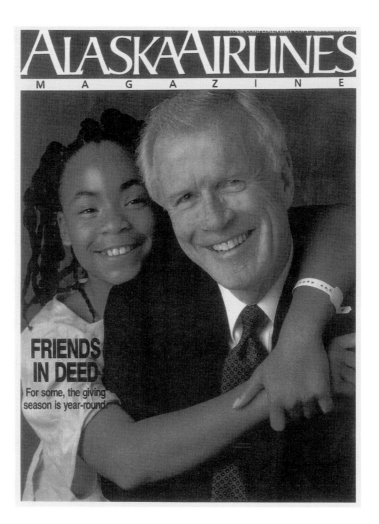

The Phone Call

And what about tomorrow, and tomorrow, and tomorrow?

First, I'm not anticipating any unexpected long-distance phone calls. I have, however, discussed with our receptionist, Diana, the possibility of a long-long-long distance phone call coming into the dealership. When or if that call comes, the conversation might well go as follows:

"And did you wish to speak with Phil Jr.?"

"No, I want to speak with Phil Sr., the old one."

"And whom may I say is calling?"

"This is the Lord calling."

Now Diana, I want you to proceed very carefully, much like this: "You are certain you wish to speak to Phil Sr?"

"Quite sure. Is he there?"

"Well, sir, I certainly mean no disrespect, but he has told me that should I ever, ever receive a phone call from you asking for him, that I was to place you on hold. He isn't through yet."

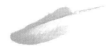

No smile is as beautiful as the one that struggles through tears.

—Unknown